GRIMETIME LIVE

(SLUM-DAWG FILTHONAIRE)

PT. III

Grimetime Live
Copyright 2015 Cavebabies press
1st edition

Excecutive editor - Randall J.C. Vargas
Excecutive proofreader - Harmony Rose
Artwork by - Paul Wesley langway III
Cover art layout - Cedric Chambers

First edition
Isbn:978 - 1511668729

Poem 52 appears in Red Fez online magazine

A special thanks to: Austin fields, Brent Tittle, Gina Tron, Nicole Hann Sullivan, Bud Smith, John Hess, Jason Hardung, Bookbar, Birdy magazine, Sam Collins, Taylor Kirk, Joe Kemp, a.razor, Thaddeus Polster, (Anna & Marleigh too) Colton McCormick, Alex Reaves, Justin Smetters, Madeline Johnston, Alana Wool, Ben Clary, Toby Krause, Stacey Marcellus, Jenstarr, Dustin Holland, Frankie Metro, Mik Longhofer, Elly Portny, Ryder Collins, Kevin Jacobs, Joe Supan, Hannah Hurrie, Joe Wallace, Hunter-Dragon Lindsey-Lou, Ben Dahlby, Michele McDonald & The Literary Underground (USA), Bookbar (CO), Cappellos (Co), Birdy Magazine (CO), Tiny-Amp Records (CO), Kleft-Jaw Press (NM), RAW-PAW (ATX), & my mother, father, Christy, Max & Sadie... & of course, The F*J*O*A

DEATH:

I retired white water

in layers of leaves.

Mountain spirits -

comfort me

52.

spruce
bringsteen my dopamine receptors to acceptable
levels
pleaseeee
assimilate fever and general anesthesia so we
wont be treated like dope fiends with amnesia
into the needless "Jesus's" needles please us, in
haste the seasons bring us
seizures
on fences
we're crucified with air tanks and dentures
slight dementia brings us to the far side
when was our apartide or do we dust not get a
garden of Eden..
pesticides.
lesions are liaisons
WHO
teach lessons as day jobs, squabble squawk with
the jealous poppy cock, take a frolic off a hill
and want not
spill your inner workings in a rainbow cataclysm
an orgasm for the culture vultures and intellectual
timberwolves
golden hooves carry me to danger.
away from these wagers
life
and the ever lasting favors
brave is never saying good bye
well at least in these eyes
because returns are intimate
and the rest is a lost cause
a brief pause in this runaway train called life
i'm married to the road
the freedom is my wife.
but away from the constant change,
or the art that is painstaking and draining
every inch of thought
creation is a form of destruction,
dismantling while assembling
the main purpose of life

isn't it to take chances and be generous?
whether that means with your feelings
or your belief system.
the name of the game is LIGHT,
LOVE

up from the

get go blast from the past/yo/robots drinking
petrol/night skies light up like the fifth of July/
the only rights is fulfillment as a weekend
warrior in disguise/reprise/the only entrepreneur
who spits crazy maneuver has you up in arms like
you was praising your fueuer/ explanations are
rural/southern head, cornbread fed/ Wu-Tang reciting
white kid from T.E.Xissss entangled in stove runs
and coastal pirate missions gets you thinking of
transcontinental condo timesharing
spare me.
the rest is baring down on me like a pyramid

with eyelids.

KOMBUCHA:

inhale smoke
exhale art
throw water balloons full of LSD at the cops.
kill barren cells with a chocolate box full of
anti-depressents for starts
repress memories all the way back from Clinton's
precedence -
lose yourself in the scatter plot
let alcohol turn tha inner monologue to brawls
in the parking lots
heaven in an everlasting DMT trip
I wish I could bring the entire planet along
sometimes you have to take the drug on a walk
stalk home-pages of your former lovers in hopes
to be a forgotten
thought.
rent out that soul of yours and throw a rave in it
dance on the graves of one million rorshachs
out foxed/out loved
blacked out in the solar system hella fucked up
off anti-biotics and LOVE

COLLABERATION IS CURRENCY:

I took a hike yesterday
it was to the center of my being.
a place where my heart bellowed
where it beat poetry unknowingly.
I had thought of showing you these
"teachings"... at least that's what they are to me.
but I didn't know if you had come yet to realize
that you are of the universe... just as me.
I wrote until these paws were raw on what I
came to see as truth
until all these made up characters came too
invoked a sense of feeling, like peeling off dreams
as you float closer to the moon.
It□s only hard because we make it so
let others greed keep our lips sewn
but I guess... if no one else is going to do anything
I'll just figure out how make this discourse bloom.
poems are only a first step to full blown love
for myself too
the ones that this course has so delicately chose
... like napping on the shore of the river before
going home because getting lost in the stream is
simply becoming one with the flow.
I feel these feelings grow, ever more sober now from
substances
I can feel the pain in my own home ... the weight
I've lost
the weight I've brought ... such is the undertow
but masterpeices can become varnished too ...a
metaphor for views
an explanation out of fear
which is the heart of love...so I grow (I hope)
if this is my last beer... MAKE IT THE STRONGEST
DRINK THERE IS
if this is my last sentence... TAKE IT FOR WHAT IT
REPRESENTS...we all have our parts to play
for each their own taste... however hellacious.

Napalm death:

GGGasoline & $tyrofoam poem|
keeps going long after we're done.
as the heat of the summer drags us to the nearest
pub...no publicity though...this is the underground
...MY HOME.
it's not often one can feel safe
all the comforts of the world at your disposal
but when you treat them like delicate morsels
the entire earth opens...and swallows you whole.
there's a hole where my head is
I'm gonna replace it with a fish-bowl
maybe then I'll have a date for the glass eyed disco
string bows & load clips while whistling all the way
home. this is equal parts gasoline & orange juice
concentrate a pinch of saw dust with soap wrapped
along the basin this is corporate art, genre
specific music 200 million dollar productions
with green screens
& cameos aching
this is the fall of western civilization
...& the dawn of a new aging
this is the plunger
and the damage done
& here I lay
high and
alone.

G XX XX SXVXX:

needles are a reoccurring theme
major cities get the best of me
seen friends fiend for spreads
speak of getting steady ... never wake up again.
dead serious when I talk on this - ish
feds bring in the dish
cartel spread the head
and the decapitated body is our
dilapidated barrios with yards full of dead.
twenties spill like sewage
fluid movements amongst the ruthless
truth is ... the fix is the spinach,
the riggers will be dead in a few years as it is.
you'll see bids from here to Tim-
bucks too, so much you'd flood the crawl space
simply because you had too ...
and that's why I turned my back to it
never slung, but everyone gets trapped in movement
distribution would have had me damn near
institutionalized
probably wouldn't have survived the first
moon cycle
rule number 5. never get high on your
own supply
but I spy a couple QT pies with some wise eyes
see if they think these QPs worth a 3 piece or more
if so ... 3.14 seconds have the dream team
at the door
couple of muffled words
then never more.
"since i got shot...my pussy game gone
through the roof"
real talks on distant sunny afternoons.

HEAVEN:

as we'd wade through clouds & lakes

switching spots (sipped sake)

we waste the day, asleep

in a field of poppies

LOOSE FITTING FUNERAL TUX:

there is no room for my error   :
yet in an era of shattered roles, I've assumed
a regalia
the smell of vagina is in the air, and I have
no more spare failures
careless,truthfull and a machine gun mouth
loaded with parables
fair is fair in a world full of failure
I've scaled interstates in search of therapy
charity is the aforementioned in veil
most stories written in fractal's paradys
insidious trips with life altering trails.
but they mean well/the kids out there in hell.
jail's a sonofabitch, I can only imagine

the department of correction.

bail.
post it. skip town. roast it
...your brain that is
collect kids like pokemon cards in your
traveling caravan of bad decisions
revelations never happen at the beginning
the universe spares for extreme moments of
unclarity.
spare me the questions of longevity,
my moral structure is true
blueprints of a revolution haunt me like a
sore tooth
yet
her energy rests in my chest, and I feel
that's the greatest taboo.
you can have it all, but will it have
you.....

MCMXCVII:

I day dream pretty women out in C I N C Y
while sailingin-between sentencingssss...

I chase C.R.E.A.M. like I was only driving saleen(z)
talk about failing, I'm so rich you can taste me...

FUCK your reply, here is my statement:
mind over maintenance
love over bank statements.
couches, Hondas & parsonages were what

I was raised in,
a toast to all these days spent waiting ...

UMmmmm/YOOOOOOOOOOOOO

I can tell you what the business is,
better yet I can limit it...
I been counting dividends/spinnin them

like synonyms

in and out of sentences

killen em relentless....shiiiiiiit

...can you tell me what a good artist izzz...

or better yet how you figure it?
I been getting grimy(ist)
rhyming, with a timing split
impeccably reenacting all these past
poetic rhetoric
& I'm flowing with the currents still ...
so much so it gives me chillllls.
on & off coasts, like he must be a fuckin' ghost
...shout out to the heads with their veins
full of hope

L O V 3:

I have three loves////
the first being the art which whips from my lungs
it gets the emotions stuck in this
throat coughed up
& hung...when I'm asleep at night...
however murky my trust... I feel like I glow...
a poet lost & rung.
I know that I grow... thats evident by the
splits in my gifts... every word sung
my second love is the hydro... so many
puns for the gigs & the shits...wits undone
the seeds I planted deep which I feel cultivate
in my soul... hung like the
stars we shine under
a breath of ephianies that couples with the words...
the pictures which
dripped from my mold... a wave from the tide
we sleep under
the third... my muse... a mermaid from the
lip of the gulf
the name of the capital city from my
childhoods state...
the state of being a child when I see her
as a saint... inane drops of rain
which form to puddles of love I sip in the shade
there is no shame in my bust...
a perfect portrait of lust...
and lush feelings from two lushes
in no rush to rust over and gush... slow moving
boats on a river of trust... art... love....
I am but a cut above... only in the sense of
knowing what it is to be humble...
what it is to have known love... loss is
but a gift in the sight of the sun.

TEMPTED BY THE CYBERNETIC SNAKECHARMER:

skull cracked open/manifesting an opus
focus/gratefully dedicated to cyberspace;
samarui type sword play
disintegrating foes in fore play while
whipping up wav. charge it to the "game"
lanes obliterated due to my Prophetic dreamscapes
/GOD - MIND/
central hardwired main frame/ 3rd eye wavvvveeee.
these docs. ache due to the sea's shake
like Parkinson's...too many years of being
punched in the face.
Its like I was born to netscape & recalculate
allocate this jaw to manuscripts/stick to the
slow pace...to keep sanity/
to keep the audience in awe
like a sweet taste, the feelings of winter
came back into fall
you couldn't pay me to share files/
it just has to be provoked in a certain way
a certain sway to the poetry I've wrote
/the way I think
like a musician who leads you to be lost in the notes
like the father, son & holy ghost all drove
home the notion of docked boats...sea-sick quotes
from lonely men who dream nothing more
then dry-land...& yet floating in the universe
is so freeing that's why this computer is my being
it encompasses my reasoning/documenting my treasons/
reminding me my time here is fleeting
just as the seasons have begun to seem.
so the ropes turn to nueces...the subtle hint
turn to gentle nuances and
the salty bastards all sold their soul for comfort...
a kind of stability they bargained for
but these cities will be laid to waste
one of the many tastes of the underground...
a good way to bare the puns.

FUCKING FOR VIRGINITY:

at the speakeasy
greasy as the cheeseburger I'm eating
feeling sleazy
about to start sneezing due to all the smoke/JEEZY
SNOW - MAN level on Mario Kart
been trying to find solid reasoning why I
should even start
ragging on mafuckas who ain't got no heart...no ears
...it's not like its an art?
you're going to die. I am too.
products of our own decisions...just letting loose
decaying organic matter
same molecular structure almost as tress
leaves signal the changing of tithes
Death-Rebirth; amongst other stylings
but just what exactly have I become?
these bags under my eyelids
designer pharmecudicals/ laptop glaring
cant I just buylove?
why does life feel so statIonary?
I always feel better when my face goes numb...
when I have to fight to stay awake
just to enjoy the high I've found shade under...
scary...
I feel I've left a number of words unsaid
but then again
I also have a few bullet points rattling in this head
traveling to find stability/fucking for virginity/
bombing for peace
instruments of a reimagined beginning
just out of reach.

NAPKIN POEM:

dumpster dive free shit
spit like I'm see sick
all this psilocybin
has hings breathing.
Feindin for reasons
turbulent seasons
dimethaltryptamine
eyes of all seeing.
Leaning on that
TEXAS - TEA
staying awake due to all the
amphetamines.
The American dream
draped in the seams
close your eyes and be baptized in confetti
all hail the war machine.

RE-BIRTH:

stream-drag me down

show me the valleys & rivers

let me take shelter in the ruins

the few allies to us sinners.

NO COPIES:

so high I can hear heaven
Gods watching televison...she smiles/looks at me
says:
"get down from there"
Impaired: the journey kicks in
I was born to die anti-climactically
after a full life of dramatics & revery set in.
A softer side of these reprieves
oh those would be her eyes
the ones I see when I close
mine...such a closed mind...
like being eighteen again.
smashing mail-boxes & eating scripts
like thin mints
fitting in by fanning the flames of kids no one
bothered to burn out with...just let them singe
I wanted to learn why I hated every instance
why all those "friends"
scoffed at the notions of this beeing
heaven

but treated hell as this almighty ending
I was already living inside of it..
like an inuit...but I was awoke from that dream.
I saw the things our DARE officers warned
we'd see.
I saw why all those PSAs were made...
why our inner cities are in such decay.
I saw it all in the machinery
lost on the railways
trying to remain irrealevent
like anything is what it seems.
I am nameless as long as you call me
BONNIE.
and from that stand point...no one can
stop me.
An outlaw...but no copy
I'd rather die
then mock another human being.

#COUCHMOBB:

I really cant find a FUCK to give

probably in this swisher wrap whos guts

lay on the table like some sort of horrible gift.
Jesus,

is this finally prose? Am I fitting in?
Can I be the hero who never needed a loan?
Can I cash in all this sin?
"Princess mononokes" on... I'm feeling

"Spirited away" ofF this blunt.

if you understand refrences, then it's been a

savage few months.

dont get your chakras in a bunch
just vibe with the hush
the rush of endorphins from the synthetic opioids

& cannibas will settle the bunch
the ground workings of an international

syndicite with no basis in the south pacific
no hunch & nasal strips...a whole lot of large

portions from low-end conglomerents...so many
ties theres no such thing as a travel expense...
but in my eyes.
& there you have it:

PERCEPTION.

a whole other level of personifying gifts...

never letting opponents get anywhere near your rim.

HUMMING TELEVISION:

I eat these souls the like roads I collect
motion to the emotionless for tolls/in retrospect,
goals is the reason I speak so comfortably
my gold is the reason I sleep so sporadically...
its like I'm lost to the battery...passionately
scribbling pageantry
as poetry...
beat me raw, baby
until my eye puffs up & I have blood dripping
from these brains
listen to me rip apart these dilettantes & Zionists,
lady
I bet your soul was born to hack into mainframe.
its like I'm one with the tragedy...like all
of these paths were forewarned...
hell & heavns philanthropies on daytime TV
more and more I word my stories like smut
making sure every back thrust, suck & fuck
is one with the form
torn vaginal walls & erectile dysfunction
lackluster assumptions about lovers I never
bothered to garner introductions from...
we just started the show.

M E T A:

ain't nothin' changed but the god damn weather

all work/all play
draped in the fre$hst "Cosby" sweaters

making love to girls who like to cos-play &

sip amoretta
Im takin dabs till I'm META

swagging the fuck out in a rented (semi-stolen)

jetta
ghostriding that bitch into a seperate

dimension altogether
cant even see inside because I'm smoking

myself into a vegetable
did I regale?

I'm focused on that payscale barettas
I wanna be the fuckin G.O.A.T.

known for blowing smoke out of mech suits

from Manilla to Valhalla
straight focused on my approach to this

locust type word play
a young scholar plagued by mistakes

that throw his vibes like a boomerang
I wanna get spun shade/shine my light so

bright it gets vaped
space so heavenly it'll make her moons quake--

I pledge to remain underground until the sun fades!

nothing but consistencey...the most glourious faze

R X V G N:

the woman I loved wears veils
of spider webs.
In our past lives, we were both dilatants
poisoned to death.
like those of the Kleft,
I reside on the tops of mountains…
ready to bathe in fountains of blood
universes of symphonic wisdom
interdimensional symbolism..visons…&
an overwhelming desire to
not give a fuccckkkk.
She said:
"You'll never be nothing"
I replied:
"*Anything…
the world is just my temporary must.."
fine wine & dark chocolate all night
pool side
GRIMETIME - LIVE…for the rest of our months…
her eyes sparkled with lust
like…what's a burger without fries?
that's how I feel with her on my bus
like a play on words
a whole theatrical show about puns…
metaphors
…though none really encompass my love.
stepping stones;
just rocks skipped along the crush.
a poem
about two lushes
rolling in the brush…
hushed from all the drinks they've drunk…
then at the zenith…
I tear the ghost out of these lungs
& fear is the lonesome sum
the thoughts it has
the braids of glass that shatters
in the shadows of stars hung

IN : SSECROI

internet
oh internet
sever your ties
from my finger tips

I need to sleep...not just smoke weed and surf

google images
I need to eat...not just listen to mixtapes

I think you're great (I really do)

but its not me...it's you

you just dont quit

I forget that the sun has essential vitamins

& minerals
tanned by the light of this laptop

I realize I need you in intervals.

but then the monitor closes

my eyes do too

phone starts exploding

vibrating.

loathing...

little to no clothing as well

a swell of emotions from this comfortable bed

I pretend is the most wonderful prison cell..

internet,oh internet,you've cast a spell!

oh whalllleeee

DARKNESS:

this pain is a muse

just as much

as it is the clue

to my wrath.

this greed is a hue

on a lurid portrait of tact-

masterful hands

in an unsavory craft.

heresay like bastions

reeking of the devil's passion

to the divine comedy

that is my path,

D E F L U E N C E:

D.I.Y & DIE

I don't really mind being a scumbag for the
rest of my life.
I guess I was born to document strife
with a firm middle finger directional to the sky.
I'll eat until I'm sick
puke//
pass out
dream tough & travel across the country again.
this isn't for "fame"
who wants to be widely recognized anymore?
the more obscure,the smaller the herd
the more fun thats in store...the more it
becomes worth.
this is my course, a courtship of sorts
a plee from the universe to breed
all sorts of rewards
some of monetary value,
knowledge
all just enriching in power...theory...
waking up to the feeling of being superior
only to realize the world doesn't respect "love"
a quick check on the bank account
...I mean...a couple checks wouldn't hurt...but
I feel like Ive been running a marathon in spurts
just trying to finish it...guts like a furnace
those last .2 miles are the ones that burn□
a subtle thought as my intentions became earnest...
every route has had some sort of destination
that Im sure of
but Im filled with hesitation & if I understood
the ins & outs of the course...
like a portrait of another world-
I cant be completely honest anymore.
I think it would only hurt the work I'm trying
to accomplish... in this modern day
NSA gauntlet
they're only looking for accomplices...&
what have I to give?
but my brethren...my sisters...
villian & vilely in this ongoing rivalry of
good and evil
modern-day dragnets on vision-quests of semblance...
down-down the cyberdelic rabbit hole
the one with toll booth as it's soul
BREAK FREE...realize YOU are the MOMENT

THE SCHEME OF THINGS:

it seems as though its here again
this doubt
the reason I ruined pens
& ventured out into the open pins,
to complain about the fences around them
excuse me as I become a mountain
impenetrable
full of bridges
I dance about them, while douching them in
 gasoline
fountains of fire sprout out of the wilderness
and I have become a titan
moving onto other continents to devour them
some sort of fabricated enlightenment
I was more lost the second I found me
weak kneed
I proceed onward to do these things I
need.
freak brief accidents put things in
perspective for
me.
Old friends beating their mothers to sleep.
its far past the point of weeping
this seeping feeling is creeping up my
steeple
my temples are poundings and feeble
so this is peace?
I wish someone would have briefed me.
countless recopies for defeat
I□m astounded I□m still standing
and bleeding.
sunsets signal an end to the day,
thats the belief anyway
so I compile my thoughts and puff away.

SCUM:

sunglasses on due to all the substances
I've dropped
literally...figuratively...losing control
of ones feet due to no sleep for a
few stops
dazed & confused...high & drunken musings on
Monday morning
commutes
trams, subways & planes⬚plain pandemonium...
pure as pain.
Watching the news over eggs & bacon
the anchors go from blasted open faces to
dancing with the stars
without a hint of indignation...
indigestion starts
like I give a shit what all the
major media outlets
fart...outnumbered...expect the
masses to starve now
I mean what's a scar when theres
Photoshop and most people are
barred out
give me xanyx or give me car alarms
busted open glass jaws with blown apart bodies:
modern art.

TENDER:

When Justin died
I lost the ability to see the future
I really don't think I ever could
but he convinced me otherwise.
I've never been able to escape that pain
just live with it day to day
a sobering reality
from such a resin stained mind.
Its hard growing up
pressing your luck
still not giving a fuck…hoping…
no: praying
…someone will love you for more then a month.
accept you for your substance love
listen to the blues you spew
view the juice you've squeezed from
that beautiful brain
you're so unafraid to lose…
this mountain town is so cold
these ounces aren't really even worth it anymore
it hard keeping a low-pro
when you sell dope…even if its "legal".

FOR ONC
E:

the pacific is bleeding
& im breathing heavier with every seizure
barometric pressure sways me like reasons
& I trust my mind a little toO sweetly...
my gut...
says sit right here
for once.
tell your story from a level head
for once.
don't succumb to your peers..
for once.
this is your home...
and the most beautiful curse are these purple
mountains that keeps those stars in your scars..
burning her eyes into portraits...
telling so many stories
and all I do is listen to our recordings
in an empty apartment
for once.
but I woke up this morning
with no fear in my heart
so this evening life restarts/
regardless of the words that flutter over our
secret mornings.

GRIEF:

Man's poetry is violence

the blood spilled on barren earth canvas

it replenishes the soil

and grows trees that are warriors.

9.0:

micro-dot scatter-plot
my mistakes had the best of me,
I bought into the system &
it stripped me of reality
/reborn
it seems as if I was incorrect on my assessment.
This life is merely a
symphony of incandescence
Orchestrated
moving parts
brain &
the heart...the universe acts as some
sort of conduit (*erm...conductor*)
simply put: it's art.
I mean there is poetry in me still
like still life's of times where I felt
alive...like a stubbed toe...or a "spent" night.
I did my best to live life "right"
but all that was left was these kites
...lost in transit...like the
transition between these
summer nights & winters hamlet.
the leaves died
the trees along with them
as I took pulls from my cannibas pipe and read
Walt Whitman...I wish my bouts were
merely those of fiction.
but all this writing is friction
fantasy and vindictive realities
played out casually
sometimes...elegantly...hell sometimes
people pay.
but I never prayed for any of these things...
I prayed for ways to eat...
for the day & night to meld effortlessly
to seperate the anxiety that is the brief & the
everlasting...the questions of ANYONE
ca actually LOVE me...
these are the things a soul kneads...
unlike the dough it so desperately covets
I feel, as if often times, the scope of my
existence isn't fully covered
I am merely a canyon, cut
by the wind, rain, sands & the hands
that formed us...

RAIN CHECK// BROKEN BRAIN:

I feel the same
like some insane
inane pain in the ass.
cra$$
I put kids on blast
simply for a good
laugh.
math
was never my strong subJect
that's why I write this shit
SCREAM IT OUT IN PUBLIC.
pubic hairs,
sweat % glares from the woman who reminds
you nothing of your mother
(thank GOD)
A couple chairs over broken backs
...bodies turn to flubber
and here I put the rubber to the pavement
pay backs a bitch
here's a couple of
rain checks...it's...GRIME TIME LIVE...
a sequel to how I met your apocalypse.

R.I.P:

turnt to the sounds of thunder
I plundered for ears.
Amast a fortune of tundra...a plot for a book
a lost cause, last chance & right hook...one
too many psychedelics
on the trail of fears.
years turned to centuries
looks bred infamy
our symmetry was reminiscent of a
symphony of baseball bats...my
cold heart burned intensely.
on the fences is what the other kids seemed
about being friends...sharing dreams
so I drew...scribbled.. and wrote reams of
paper until I reached my first plateau of being
cut-class & smoked grass with the re-deem team
shepparding fiends beams of light/scenes
in deep purple nights
scattered my mind until it fell under
scrutiny of the seeing...if I could
show what's been breeding...no...that's why
I write...
every evening...
because we're all slowly dying..

SWINGSETS AT SUNRISE:

Today,
I will snip open my cerebellum
exposing the Technicolor blood that flows
let it gurgle and blurp itself into a poem.
these feelings are unknown
even to myself
I feel like my energy sweeps me through streets,
rocks me to sleep, such cheap beliefs...

that these dreams are my highway to
greater things...so I always roam.
but the writings in the wind
and it blesses me when it chooses too.
the truth is my long in the tooth attitude
is a bat of the eye to the noose...
I am not afraid to die for what I
believe is truth
that all living things are created equal/&
deserve to be treated as such
for my skin and bones is earth & stardust
which is why I speak in blizzards,
with a brushfire of love in my lungs.
hung on the thoughts of helping my fellow
brothers/sisters
I swing gently on the park swings at sunrise
over the gentle ripples of the lake,
I see the geese gulp water like wine
& think to myself
"what a hell of a time I chose to be born"

CLARITY:

Prayer by a rocky shore

eye of the storm, boats unmoored

-such is our condition.

R E A C H:

hot mess
blessed by aggressive tendencies &
an illogical anatomy
sprinkle in some agoraphobic actions
and it leads me to reading to you as
you lay in bed...
sleeping.
In hopes that some divine being/
otherworldly creature
sees me and takes notice
restores hope in this feeble preacher
because I am simply breathing□being
lead by the seasons bleeding.
asleep in the chapel
another chapter in this book of life
with converse mastodons
& sabertooths battling a galaxy/
I am but an analogy to the way things
die.

ON POINT:

Alone
atop a mountain fortress
I feel blessed to be this
fortunate... lessons so bountifull
sound waves pull me through
space time continuum
I obtain what I receive as...
allowance...a bounty from this abundant universe.
whats worse is
verse after verse
my mind goes loose into her purse
as she speaks of Versaci
such a versatile word.
I feel well versed, yet reserved
in this hollowed out
earth
eating breakfast at a diner in a
foggy metropolitan world.
but this is not the
worst thing I could have
imagined
at least I can smoke cannabis from my
porch
& the 17 year olds on hood patrol aren□t
THAT bout it, 'bout it...
murmurs from the underworld
a memoir I□ll mumble through
I feel like a bumblebee, after
leaving the earth will simply ask
"what will I do"
I hope I end up on some distant moon
in a galaxy far away
where logic & reason are praised
and ignorance is for but a few
oh...you
audience...reader
I hope you can feel this
truth.
so long in the tooth
& futile this
moot point is
...but at tmes it feels
like it's the only thing
I was born to tell you.

PYRAMID:

precise on the pavement with chalk outlines of
my neighbors scattering
it's physique.
I stapled my dreams to a chainsaw kite that cut through
the logs and limbs of my trees who themselves hung over
the ground and amongst the steeples and air traffic
control towers of my street.
Though I had never been outside before I had felt
tonight was the one where I should be.
and maybe as beautiful as it was I had only four
requests for the world
and three were to be in Rome by this evening; alas,
though, I spun
and wasted in this grave I've dug my lonesome
with bad words and pharmaceutical love songs
Constantly stumbling around questioning for
the best pint in Travis county.
I sat down at the corner of my street
so far from home
but so close to where I once knew I thought
I should have believed where I needed to be
so here I am
comfortable and still wishing
I was in Napels or pompei...anywhere close to knowledge
but truly not understanding how to learn
but with a full grasp of the road..
a question arose
as I nomad who wished not to be known
only by a few but by the unknown
and by the unknown I mean one
and by the one I mean a symphony of sight
smells and senses
relishing and tickling my inner joy be not
just a rose petal at my window
but the door to opening my world
the roots to my tree which I've chopped
down to build rafts to the sea
only to get to home which has been here all along
you & me

MANDOLIN:

I thought the days were getting shorter
really, the pain was becoming less
its like those mornings when you wake up
to thunder & lightning is when you're at your best.
I think its an underestimation of manifestations
life
sometimes the wall is set so high
like the mind could even believe in such a trial.
I think its the positioning of the sun
the sum of all fears
the pile drivers
or the years that turn into miles...or tears...
or stories
(much like this one here)
on a greyhound,
madlib & j.dilla my only companionship
I dream of championships
& chateaus with a terrace.
I used to be embarrassed about the poems I wrote
little did I know they□d be the baby step
to propelling me
where I was destined to
grow.
Below this aging exterior
sits a child who feels alone
mostly he smiles
mostly he roams.
Beautiful shades of blue
nights where the jazz were the only thoughts we'd amuse
a symphony of peril, this American dialogue
like clues to the cluster of stars where this
sabbatical started..

KRAING-PLUNGE:

your nostalgia is a drug
a tree for you to rest under
the future is mine
another syringe for me to plunder
plung deep in to the thunder
feel the grief in this spacetime - it's abundent
scumlord spitting brain bugs on the tumblr
it's only every once in a while I get long
in the numbness
spewed words run lurid with the months bend
like a horrid scene baptized in blood &
adapted for the big screen
so ruthless even it gets deemed NC-17,
never even scheduled for release.
but in the backdrop of my heart there are
always private screenings
it seems as if I'am always screaming
eternally I mean
like I want to kiss you everytime we speak
break the padlocks to the abandoned
museums and just sleep....
feel like art for an evening
I think you feel like what I've been feeling
but I don't think its right yet
so I sit down and write until I shine light
out of these eyelids...
I think its something that you said
"we're all learning how to be mindless"
I think I'm learning how to grind, kid
getting grimetime live and shining slime
through each one of my time sigs
big wig tips with a small town spirit just trying
 to get lit & fit in
between your mind,thighs &
appointments...a poet at wits end.

SMILELUST:

the quietness simmers

like a glimmer of hope, the wind whips up
and around the building again

I remember being older...bolder

thinner...so strung out on lonliness &
a general unwillingness to cope

with the things that I perceived to be out of my control.

I wanted to watch time bend

feel that I had a soul and that it was above
all worth living in
lose or gain it all on the roll of the dice
single splices of time spent that were meant
to spice up my style
but alas I am guile...
a lone wolf caught up on the thoughts of truth...

& being so in love with my youth

I sized up my rivals
cleaned up my rifle

started pile driving the cement with my fists...
using the broken fingers as ink pens

writing sonnets to the one woman I'm in love with

& to the planet I was born in

I think I became sharp in the tooth

cool,calm & collected in my blues

lifted up by my greens...but is this all
truley usefull?

all this museful meanderings...hollow panderings

eyes towards the clues...
I just want to love and to be loved back...

small hopes for a drunken fool

SOMA:

to me it seems...to question is to be free
..in sentence fragments I speak
thus
this paradox has begun to lay siege
no further theories.
delete,delete,delete!
this full head tells tales of sacred scripts so
parallel with deceit
programming spars with creation and its never as
clean as it should be...
hearts are so dug into the speech but
my love is for all...
and to not be chained to one belief...
in this sense I have tasted defeat..
and the humor I mask it with is more then fear
it's whole...of sound body and soul
an astral plateau forged of diamond
& gold.
theorize all you fear.

(death is the birth)

UNNAMED:

quiet weeping from my best friend's mother
at his wake...
"get over it"
get on top of it...
that mountain I mean...
its where the fountain of knowledge is but a stream...
drink from it...
wash yourself clean.
I used to drink-
until I fell asleep.
now I just
smoke...and everything I speak...is sad
because you aren't with me.
and I mean this in so many ways
so many...
I just wish you the best in
heaven...or hell...or purgatory...
or I hope you were reincarnated into a dragon
...and I hope you know what you meant to me...
to us
to your brothers...I just wish I could hug your mom and
tell her that it's over...and your gone...
and we can all stop crying now
but its too hard...and it isn't...and I haven't...
and I probably
wont...
I dedicated my first book to your memory
and I dedicate every 1st & 15th to your energy
& even if its a fleeting tremor
my earth is still rattled by missing you...or ye...
shit you know just as much as you,
I was always one for rhyming
I□m still climbing out of the depths of my soul
from that one day where you went home...
and I was the last to say: "goodbye, i'll see you soon."
with...or without knowing...

THERE'S POWDER ALL OVER EVERYTHING

there's powder all over everything
the ground is levitating
I've sprouted horns
thorny rose bushes encase these palms as I
stare down movie star wet dreams
the moab desert would castrate before
we saw anything
strong words for a plot boss with no cause j
ust paid by the hour,
ten pyramids to a dollar bill totem pole
scower the city for another powder
puff muff diver
ill be sky high by 8am, wandering around
flea markets in the upper saint clair
township of north Pittsburgh, Pennsylvania
smoking Marlboro menthols while I scratch my
nostrils because of recent deposits
I think its the VHS tapes, or the N64 games,
or the 3 foot bong rips
because this lifestyles getting more outrages
I've been living on TV dinners and skinned knee
antics, and placebo cream & artificial sugar cakes
black water southern rituals not for the weak
stomached individuals
mixed media stencils
that are so ritualistic its rude to
compare anything to them
for the simple fact that lightning strikes
the temple of a hardworking middle-class
man
ruptured spleen in a hospital bed, and I'm doing this
"I fell down some stairs"

(clears throat)

falling asleep in a past life
I was as honest as a Denver man can be
with half a brain,
a room key
and a whole ki
a nation of pirates who we ride with who
sleeps in your city streets
dirty, dusty and on small doses of what ever
our heads need at the moment
no chromotosing
you'll never wish to live so long....
beards growing and your listening to the same dead song
day
after
day --because its the only alone time you can ever get...
blessed be the boy who comes in ragged clothes!
scripture doesn't even do it for me anymore!
i've stared down the lord and the devil and
i've breathed a thunderous roar!
boats exploded down in the river quarry and
the sun quickly was
drowned by the storms
summers lonely blues
dark purple hearts of tours

random acts of heroism
noses full of heroin
& I'm near and trembling...
close to the moons radiant glow ripe
with anticipation and hope
the night won't be like most...
the next smile may come with tears
it's hard not to be yourself out here
city streets...
city lights.

www.ingramcontent.com/pod-product-compliance
Lightning Source LLC
Chambersburg PA
CBHW021417170526
45164CB00002B/681

9781511668729